Overcoming Illness & Disease Through Juicing

By
Fred L. Gist

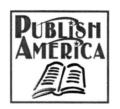

PublishAmerica
Baltimore

Hardcover 9781462649419
PUBLISHED BY PUBLISHAMERICA, LLLP
www.publishamerica.com
Baltimore

Printed in the United States of America

FOREWORD

This book is not meant to treat or cure any ailment or life threatening disease. The recommendations in this book can help you see results. Juice on a daily basis 32-64 ounces of juice. Follow the juice mixtures in this book and you will see results. Also be sure to drink the juice mixtures shortly after you make them! May this book be a blessing too you.

CONTENTS

INTRODUCTION 5

WHAT IS JUICING 7

WHY JUICE AND THE BENEFITS 8

FRESH JUICE VERSES PASTEURIZED JUICE 9

CONFIRMING DATA 11

IMPORTANT DEFINITIONS 12

FRUITS AND VEGETABLES, THEIR THERAPEUTIC

BENEFITS 15

ABOUT THE AUTHOR 47

FINAL THOUGHTS 49

4 THINGS TO HELP YOU LIVE LONGER 50

REFERENCES 51

CHANGE YOUR EATING HABITS TO BECOME WELL

AGAIN...52

WASHING YOUR ORGANIC FRUITS AND

VEGETABLES 53

BENEFITS OF USING A JUICER....................................54

WHAT JUICER DO I USE..55

INTRODUCTION

Juicing is a powerful process of vital importance in improving your overall health. Juicing will also boost your immune system and give you more energy to fight off disease. Juicing will get rid of and eliminate harmful toxins from your body.

The vitamins and minerals in the juicing process are very beneficial. Juicing lowers blood pressure, contributes to better overall cardiovascular health, increases your physical performance, gives you much more energy and helps you sleep better.

(Genesis 1:29) Fruits and vegetables have been recognized from the beginning as a powerful natural source of important nutrients very essential to our health, even in the beginning in the Garden of Eden.

We can drink much more juice than we could ever eat whole fruits and vegetables. When you separate the fiber from the juice you gain much of the nutritional value and benefit simply by drinking a glass of juice. The juice also has a higher concentration of minerals, vitamins, enzymes, and trace elements that build strong healthy cells. When you drink freshly extracted juices on a daily basis you are now doing daily "Juice Therapy." This nutritionally "Juice Therapy" can and will revitalize your cells, in an amazingly short period of time. "Juice Therapy," drinking raw juices is the healthiest thing you can do for your body!

Today many of our physical bodies, especially here in the western world have degenerated very seriously. The reason is we have been trying to build new cells in our body with dead and toxic building materials. We can renew this hope, even if these cells have advanced deterioration. Raw fruit and vegetable juices are a source of superior building materials.

If we provide our bodies with these superior building materials we then build new cells, and these new cells will be superior in nature. These new cells will be stronger and healthier than the cells they are replacing. In these raw fruits and vegetables are the plant chemicals called Phytochemicals.

These Phytochemicals are the key in preventing cancer, heart disease, arthritis and other ailments and disease. I invite you, I urge you to start drinking these healing juices.

WHAT IS JUICING

Juicing removes separates out the fiber. These juices are then quickly digested into the body in a very short period of time. (minutes) You will then receive much more of the nutritional benefits of the fruits and vegetables, and by drinking the juice it will be the healthiest thing you can do for your body.

You receive in juicing vitamins, minerals, the trace elements, and enzymes in their most concentrated and natural form. The body puts these juices to work without long digestion time, and your body is receiving "Live Food". This "Live Food" will make you feel, look better and become healthier. Raw juice has a laxative effect (more evident in fruit juices) which helps to rid your body of toxins. By extracting the juice from fruits and vegetables and then drinking it immediately you then feed your cells.

Nutrients are contained, locked up in fruits and vegetables in the liquids and held together by the fiber and the skin. So the nutrients are in the liquid not the fiber.

WHY JUICE AND THE BENEFITS

When you extract the fiber from the juice you are eliminating the liquid from the fiber and you are supplying your body with life giving nutrients. Your body is then receiving the maximum amount of these nutrients. This fresh life giving, healing juice, is not pasteurized it is free of preservatives and additives. It is fresh pure juice. It is not like supermarket juices that are bottled, canned and cooked. (pasteurized) This cooked (pasteurized) process results in dead food, which means all the nutrients are killed.

The juices of raw fruits and vegetables are the richest sources of vitamins and minerals and their trace elements that can be found. Fresh juices are also "Alkaline" which neutralizes all the "Acids" in the body. Acids create aliments and disease. If we eat too much "Meat" it produces acids. This then causes different kinds of ailments and diseases.

Fruit juices are the cleansers of the human body, and vegetable juices are the builders of the human body. By juicing fruits and vegetables we gain many nutritional benefits. You can then literally juice your way to maximum health when you combine different types of fruits and vegetables on a daily basis, then this assures that your body receives its full quota of vitamins and minerals.

FRESH JUICE VERSES PASTEURIZED JUICE

When you juice fresh (Organic) fruits and vegetables you add to your body life healing nutrients, enzymes, minerals, antioxidants, vitamins, phytochemicals, and chlorophyll just to name a few. I haven't said it before but I must stress that it is very important to juice only "Organic" fruits and vegetables.

These "Organic" fruits and vegetables are free of pesticides which means they are produced without the use of these pesticides and synthetic fertilizers, genetic engineering, growth hormones, sewer sludge fertilizers, antibiotics and irradiation. I read an article in a health magazine not long ago that every time we eat non Organic fruits and vegetables that we are ingesting several different types of pesticides.

The nutrients that you make from your own juice are far more superior and powerful than anything you buy in a carton, can, or bottle from a local supermarket. These packaged juices are diluted with water. There are additives, preservatives included that suppress the potency of the fruits and vegetables. Chemicals are included which destroy the nutrients. These juices are also heated to high temperatures as part of the pasteurization process, which only prolongs their shelf life. This pasteurization process then kills the life giving enzymes. Fresh "Organic" juice is the only way to get these life giving enzymes, antioxidants, minerals, vitamins, phytochemicals, nutrients, and trace elements.

A glass of healthful juice quickly puts vitamins and minerals into your bloodstream. When you juice "Organic" fruits and vegetables you maximize available vitamins and minerals found in these "Organic" fruits and vegetables. When you drink fresh juice mixtures on a daily basis it provides an important health benefit. It gives you nutrients lost in your normal daily living.

Vitamins have properties that benefit the human body. The vitamins found in these "Organic" fruits and vegetables reduce the risk of heart disease, cancers, muscular degeneration of the eyes in the elderly, stroke, and nerve damage.

CONFIRMING DATA

Medical doctor Max Gerson put 50 cancer patients on a juice regimen. It is described in detail in his book "A Cancer Therapy:" results of Fifty Cases. All 50 people he discussed recovered from cancer through natural treatments. Dr. Bircher-Bonner found the same results working with many of his patients. He found that green juice was very therapeutic.

Dr. Norman W. Walker recovered from illness by eating a raw food and juice diet. Dr. Walker lived to be a ripe old age of 109 years old. Many people got well through his program also. The original "Juice Man" Jay Kordich recovered from a life threatening cancer through a daily regimen of carrot and apple juice. Dr. George Malkmus the founder of Hallelujah Acres was diagnosed with advanced stage melanoma cancer.

Dr. Malkmus completely recovered through a raw food and juicing program. This is a few names of people who have become well again because of the power of juicing. The enzymes, vitamins, minerals in the juice promote healing and give you protection from disease. Juice therapy has helped thousands of people recover from life threatening illness.

IMPORTANT DEFINITIONS

Nutrients = Substances needed by the body to maintain health and life. These are the vitamins and minerals present in the fruits and vegetables.

Beta Carotene = A substance that the body uses to produce vitamin A. Carrot juice contains large quantities of vitamin A in the form of Beta Carotene. Beta Carotene is an antioxidant that helps the body detoxify. Beta Carotene is an antioxidant that has demonstrated powerful abilities to inhibit rapid production of new cancer cells. It also lowers the risk of heart disease, increased immunity and gives us better mental functioning.

Vitamins = Fruits and Vegetables are excellent sources of many vitamins. Vitamins are needed for tissue maintenance and normal growth. Vitamins are essential for life and health. Many vitamins cannot be manufactured by our bodies, thus need to be supplied. Vitamins are complex substances that are essential to good health. Juicing is a natural and easy way to ensure that your daily intake of necessary vitamins is met.

Free Radicals = Free Radicals are small molecules with an extra electron. It is highly chemically reactive. Free Radicals attack cells and cause a lot of damage in the body. Free Radicals damage our DNA codes in the nucleus of the cell. Free Radicals are highly unstable compounds that attack our cell membranes causing cell breakdown, aging and a predisposition to some diseases. Free Radicals result from air pollution, smoking, heated fats and oils among just a few things.

Antioxidants = Minerals, Vitamins, Enzymes, and Anutrient compounds. Antioxidants are substances that block and inhibit destructive damage to your cells. Antioxidants are compounds that protect our cells by preventing polyunsaturated fatty acids in cell membranes from oxidizing thus neutralizing Free Radicals. Antioxidants are fully found in fruits and vegetables. These Antioxidants counteract "Free Radicals" that cause cellular damage. Antioxidants protect your cells by carrying "Free Radicals" out of your body. Vitamins C,E and Beta Carotene are high in Antioxidant properties.

Anutrients= Compounds that protect the body from the environment. Anutrients are found in fruits, vegetables and grains. Anutrients are also the pigments such as the carotenes (yellow, red) the Chlorophylls (green), the Anthocyanins (red, blue), the Proanthocyanidins (colorless), and the flavonoids (colorless or yellow).

Minerals= Inorganic elements in its simpliest form that is required by the body. Major minerals are Potassium, Sulfur, Magnesium, Sodium, Chloride, Phosphorus, and Calcium. Minerals are found in our fruits and vegetables and are essential for optimum health.

Enzymes= Enzymes are protein, organic catalysts which speed chemical reactions in the body, thus breaking down and absorbing foods quicker in our body. Enzymes are found in fruits and vegetables.

Phytochemicals= Phytochemicals are plant chemicals found in fruits and vegetables. Phytochemicals protect against cancer, heart disease and are keys in preventing these and some of our most deadly diseases. Phytochemicals have various health promoting properties. Phyto is a Greek word which means to bring forth, a prefix meaning from a plant.

There are many fruits and vegetables that can be juiced. You can juice many in different combinations. I am listing fruits and vegetables that are the most important ones to juice, because of their greater health benefits. I am also including juicing combinations of other fruits and vegetables that will be very beneficial to your health. It is important again to only juice "Organic" fruits and vegetables, because they are free of pesticides.

FRUITS AND VEGETABLES, THEIR THERAPEUTIC BENEFITS

ALFALFA= Great source of Chlorophyll. Good for wounds, burns, Arthritis, Rheumatism, Gout. Helps improve the bodies resistance to cancer, reduces inflammation, lowers Cholesterol levels.

APPLE= An Immune system booster. Good for the digestive track. Liver stimulant, laxative, direuretic, lowers Cholesterol, keeps blood glucose levels up. Vitamins A,C,B,G and Beta Carotene. Key ingredient is "Pectin" which can lower risk of Colon cancer. Also contains Boron which is good to help prevent Calcium loss which leads to Osteoporis. Good for Menopausal women, because it boosts blood levels of the hormone Estrogen. Minerals= Calcium, Magnesium, Phosphorus, Potassium, Copper, Zinc. Juice Apple, remove seeds.

ARTICHOKE= Lowers Cholesterol, Cleanser for the Liver, diuretic. Good for the Pancreas, Spleen. Maintains normal blood sugar levels. Minerals are Phosphorus, Magnesium, Potassium, Folic acid, Sodium, Beta Carotene. Vitamins are B3 and Vitamin C. Juice the entire plant.

ASPARAGUS= Promotes healing, antioxidant, anti-cancer, anti-cataracts, diuretic, rich in Vitamin E. It is a good source of Vitamin C and A. Minerals are Niacin, Potassium and Iron. Juice the entire plant.

BEET= High in Vitamin A and Betaine and enzyme that strengthens and nourishes the Liver. Contains Chlorine which cleanses the Liver, Kidney and Gall Bladder. Beets are a good source of Potassium. Beets are good for pregnant women, because they provide high levels of Folate, which can reduce the risk of Spina Bifida in unborn children. The minerals that are found in Beets are Calcium, Phosphorus, Iron, Potassium, and Sodium. Beets also contain Sulfur which has been known to treat and help prevent tumors. Juice leaves, Beet and root.

BLUEBERRIES= Great source of Vitamin C, Pectin, and Potassium. Blueberries are a great antioxidant. They are anti-bacterial and anti-viral. Blueberries contain Tannins which kill bacteria and viruses. Blueberries are good for Bladder infections and high Cholesterol. Juice all.

BROCCOLI= Broccoli is rich in Phytonutrients which help to fight cancers. Broccoli is an antioxidant, it is anti-cancer, anti-cataract and it promotes healing. Broccoli is high in Vitamin C, high in Indoles, Glucosinolates and Dithiolthiones, known for their cancer fighting properties. Broccoli is also rich in Folate, Beta Carotene, Vitamin C, Iron, and Potassium. Juice stalks to get juice content.

BRUSSEL SPROUTS= Brussel Sprouts are good for the Pancreas. They are the highest producer of Folate necessary for the production of white blood cells. Brussel Sprouts are in rich in Potassium, Vitamin C, Folate, and Beta Carotene. It is a close relative of the Cabbage.

CABBAGE= The Cabbage is good for stomach ulcers, heart disease, and cancer. Is is a good source of Vitamin C, Beta Carotene and Folate. Dr. Max Gerson, M.D. put 50 of his cancer patients on a Cabbage juice regimen. His book is "A Cancer Therapy: Results of Fifty Cases. All 50 people recovered. The Cabbage is anti-ulcer, anti-inflammatory, diuretic, anti-cataract, promoting healing, anti-cancer, and immune builder and anti-bacterial. Cabbage is high in cancer fighting Endoles. Cabbage is a good source of Choline. It is high in Vitamin E. Cabbage is good for the Liver, and is effective in preventing colon cancer. Cabbage reduces blood sugar in diabetics and is effective in preventing and healing ulcers. Sauer Kraut juice which is the juice of the Cabbage contains lactic acid that is very soothing for your intestines. It is good for the gastrointestinal tract.

Dr. Lee W. Wattenburg of the Department of Laboratory Medicine and Pathology at the University of Minnesota in Minneapolis published an article in the May 1978 issue about Cancer research. (38:1410-13) It showed that Brussel Sprouts, Cabbage, Cauliflower, and Broccoli inhibit the development of harmful chemical carcinogens within the body. Dr. Donald R. German recommended Sulfur rich vegetables in his book, the Anti-Cancer Diet (New York, Wideview Books, 1980) Brussel Sprouts, Cabbage, Broccoli, Cauliflower, Spinach, Turnips, Lettuce, Celery, and Dill. Juice all of the Cabbage, except the hard bottom core.

CANTALOUPE= Cantaloupes are great blood thinners, thus decreasing the risk of heart attacks and strokes. Cantaloupes also reduce the risk of cancer. Cantaloupes are a good source of Vitamin A, Vitamin C, and Calcium. Cantaloupe is a great antioxidant and is anti-cancer. Juice all, rind included!

CARROTS= Carrots lower blood Cholesterol, Carrots are anti-bacterial, an immune booster, anti-cancer, antiseptic, antioxidant, artery protecting, and extremely nutritious. Carrots are rich in Vitamin A, B, and C. The minerals found in Carrots are Iron, Calcium, Potassium and Sodium. Carrots clean the Liver and digestive track. Carrots help prevent kidney stones and relieves gout and arthritis. The Beta Carotene in Carrots cut cancer risks. Carrots also protect you from heart disease. Carrots promote mental functioning and decrease the risk of cataracts.

CARROTS are the sweetest of the vegetables. If you are a diabetic you need to mix in three fourths more greens (Spinach

, *Parsley) to reduce the sugar content. Carrots are good for heartburn and they protect you from cancer of the mouth and rectum. Juice the Carrot, but remove the greens and cut of the top of the Carrot.*

CELERY= Celery is good for gout and urinary infections. Celery reduces inflammation in arthritis sufferers. Juice all.

CHERRY= Cherries boost the immune system, because they contain powerful antioxidants. Cherries are rich in Vitamin C, Beta Carotene, Folic Acid, Calcium, Magnesium, Phosphorus, Potassium, Biotin and Flavonoids. Please remove seeds when juicing. They can destroy your juicer!

CRANBERRY= Cranberries are great for urinary tract infections, like cystitis. Cranberries are anti-cancer, anti-bacterial, anti-viral and are a great antioxidant. Cranberries keep bacteria from attaching to the walls of the urinary tract. Remove seeds.

ELDERBERRY= Elderberries have twice the antioxidant power of blueberries and more than 50% antioxidant power of cranberries. Elderberries are called the fruit of the American Elder. Elderberries are an effective antioxidant for arthritis. The Elderberry is very similar to the grape. It is higher in Vitamin C, Niacin, and protein. The Elderberry has bioflavonoids that improve circulation and strengthen blood vessels. The Elderberry is great to treat colds and the flu, because it destroys the ability of viruses to infect a cell.

Elderberries have antioxidant properties that are useful in the treatment of cancer. Elderberries help lower cholesterol, improve vision, improves your heart health, and boosts your immune system. Elderberries are good for asthma, bronchitis, HIV, and reduces inflammation of the urinary tract and Bladder. The Elderberries unique proteins regulate the immune system helping the body defend against disease.

GARLIC= Garlic is great for fighting infections like colds. Studies have shown that Garlic prevents the formation of cancer cells. Garlic reduces the risk of blocked arteries and heart disease. Garlic protects organs from radiation, and chemical pollutants. Garlic lowers Cholesterol, stimulates the appetite, dissolves mucus in the sinus cavities, bronchial tubes and the lungs. Garlic gets rid of intestinal parasites. Garlic lowers blood sugar and is rich in Potassium, Calcium and Magnesium. Juice all.

GRAPE= Grapes fight carcinogens. (any substance that produces cancer) Grapes are good for arthritis, the urinary tract and Grapes lower blood pressure. Grapes protect the heart, are anti-cancer because they contain Ellagic Acid the Phytonutrient which helps deplete cancer in the body. Grapes are a good source of Potassium, Fructose, Glucose, and Vitamin C. ("The Grape Cure," Johanna Brandt)

KALE= Kale is very high in Calcium. Kale is great for osteoporosis and Calcium deficiencies. It is important to know that "Vegetable Calcium" in Kale, Broccoli, Bok Choy, Turnips Collards, and Mustard Greens is absorbed in higher quantities than milk. Kale benefits the nerves, kidneys, muscles, skin, blood and heart. Kale is high in Vitamin A which is a great benefit to the teeth, soft tissue, hair and eyes. Kale stimulates the immune system and is rich in Beta Carotene, Folate, Calcium and Potassium.

LEMON= The Lemon is a diuretic and is good for coughs, colds, and the flu. Lemons are rich in Vitamin C, Potassium, Fructose, and Calcium. Juice the whole Lemon, remove the seeds. Juice the skin also. *The Lemon adds flavor/zest to other juices.

LETTUCE= Lettuce is rich in Vitamin A,C,Calcium, Iron, Folic Acid, Potassium, and Chlorophyll. Lettuce is an antioxidant and is anti-cancer. Collard Greens, Chard, Kale, Mustard and Turnip Greens have the same properties as Lettuce. Lettuce and these are greens keep the colon healthy. Lettuce can be good for pregnant women to help protect against Spina Bifida. Lettuce is rich in Iron and Magnesium. Lettuce is a great diuretic. Lettuce is good for infants because of its Iron content. Juice all.

ORANGE= The Orange is high in anti-cancer properties. The Orange is high in Vitamin C, Potassium, Lutein, and Carotene. Oranges are great for colds and Oranges lower Cholesterol. Oranges are high in Limonene which inhibits Breast Cancer. Oranges are a good source of Choline. Oranges contain Flaavonoids, Coumarins, Limonoids, Terpenes, and Carotenoids, which make it along with other Citrus Fruits a strong cancer fighter. Remove peel and seeds when juicing.

PARSLEY= Parsley is rich in Vitamin C, contains Vitamin A, Potassium, Magnesium, Iron, Phosphorus, Calcium, and Sodium. Parsley is good for the kidneys, skin infections, the Thyroid, blood vessels, the eyes and menstrual cramps. It is a good to combine Parsley with Carrot Juice, with more Carrot juice than Parsley.

PARSNIP= Parsnip is good for cleansing the Liver and Gall Bladder. Parsnip is good for kidney stones. Parsnips are anti-cancer and anti-inflammatory. Parsnips are good sources of Niacin, Vitamin C, Vitamin B, Vitamin E, Folate and Potassium. Parsnips contain some Calcium and Iron. Mix with Carrot Juice. Remove tops.

PINEAPPLE= Pineapple is rich in Beta Carotene, Vitamin C, Potassium and Bromelain. Bromelain is good for digestion and good for blood clots. Pineapple is a great sweetner. I mix it with Carrot juice and other green juices such as Parsley, and Spinach. I also add an apple. It makes a great tasting juice. Always remove the outer green core.

POTATOES (WHITE)= White Potatoes are good for reducing the risk of heart disease. White Potatoes are good for treating Lung Cancer and skin blemishes. Combine White Potatoes with Carrot juice. White Potatoes are good for cleansing the entire system. White Potatoes are good for gout and sciatica. *For Gout mix one pint of equal parts of Beet, Cucumber and Carrot and juice daily. *To see good results you must eliminate meat, chicken and fish. White Potatoes are rich in Calcium, Vitamin C, Carotenes, Fiber, Folate, and Potassium. Juice all.

POTATOES (SWEET)= Sweet Potatoes contain much more Calcium than White Potatoes.(3 times) Sweet Potatoes contain 2 times more Sodium, 2 times more Silicon, and 4 times more Chlorine than Potatoes.(White) Sweet Potatoes are very helpful in protecting against cancers. Sweet Potatoes are rich in Vitamin E,C, and Beta Carotene. Juice all.

RADISH= Radishes are good for sinus problems, relieves mucus problems and decreases risk of Stomach and Lung cancers. Radishes are good sources of Calcium, Folate, Iron, Vitamin A, C, Magnesium, Phosphorus, and Potassium. Radishes are good for the Thyroid and are good for constipation. I suggest you mix Radish juice with Carrot juice. It is to strong to drink alone. Juice all.

RED GRAPEFRUIT= Red Grapefruit is high in cancer fighting Lycopene. Red Grapefruit protects strongly against Colon and Stomach cancer. Red Grapefruit is good for the eyes. Red Grapefruit aids in digestion. Red Grapefruit is rich in Potassium, Folate, Calcium, and Vitamin C. Remove skin and seeds.

SPINACH= Spinach is good for osteoporosis. Spinach is a great detoxifier and is good for anemia because of its Iron content. Spinach is good for fatigue especially during Female *monthly periods. (mix with Carrot juice) Spinach is good for constipation and is a cleanser and healer for the entire intestinal tract. Spinach is good for lowering blood pressure, good for arthritis, anemia, nerves, headaches.(including migraines) Spinach is rich in Iron, Beta Carotene, Calcium and Folate. Mix with Carrot juice. Wash to remove dirt. Juice all.*

STRAWBERRY= Strawberries are good for arthritis, gout, rheumatism, the Liver and kidney stones. Strawberries are high in cancer fighting Ellagic Acid and Vitamin C. Strawberries are anti-cancer, and antioxidant and anti-viral. Strawberries are also high in Vitamin C, Calcium, Magnesium, Phosphorus, and Potassium. Strawberries are a great sweetener. Juice all. Juice the firmest strawberries.

STRING BEANS= String Beans are great for Diabetics because it contains ingredients that produce natural insulin. Combine String Bean juice with Carrot juice. Drink (2) pints daily. Juice all.

TOMATO= Tomatoes lower the risk of many cancers and help prevent heart disease. Tomatoes contain Lycopene a powerful antioxidant. Tomatoes are rich in Vitamin C, Beta Carotene, Potassium, Folate and Lycopene. Tomatoes are high in Glutathione. Tomatoes are also good for the kidneys. Juice all.

WATERMELON= Watermelon is good for skin problems, arthritis, gout, fevers, headaches and sour stomach. Watermelon is a great diuretic, detoxing and antioxidant. Watermelons regenerate the blood because acid is flushed from the system. Watermelons are rich in Calcium, Vitamin C, B5, Folic Acid, Phosphorus, Potassium and Beta Carotene. Watermelons contain Vitamin A, C, Iron and Potassium. The seeds of the Watermelon contain Vitamin E and Zinc.

Watermelons are anti-cancer and anti-bacteria. Juice all including the rind. The rind contain many healing properties, just like the Cantaloupe. (The good stuff)

WHEAT GRASS= Wheat Grass juice is anti-cancer, it cleanses the blood, it is an antibiotic, it protects against radiation and is anti-inflammatory. Wheat Grass contains a powerful healing agent called Chlorophyll. It's also a powerful infection fighter which is high in Vitamin C, E and Beta carotene. You really need to buy a Wheat Grass juicer but if you don't, do what I use to do. I would wrap the Wheat Grass in bunch of Spinach and then push it through with a large Carrot. It works. The Wheat Grass juice is dispensed!

The following pages will give you juice combinations for different ailments. It is important to use only "Organic" fruits and vegetables. Organic means that these fruits and vegetables have not been treated with any type of harmful pesticide. I'm also including my "Special Bonus Section" following these juice combinations.

Immune Booster

(6) Carrots
(1) Half Beet
(4) Broccoli Stems
(2) Large Chunks Pineapple

Fights infection, bacteria, and other viruses

Detox Kooler

(3) Carrots
(1) Half Watermelon Rind
(1) Half Watermelon
(8) Strawberries
Juice the skin/rind of the watermelon it's full of antioxidants.

This is a great way to detoxify your body. This drink is rich in Vitamin C, E, Beta Carotene, Potassium, and Zinc. It flushes your body and helps it fight bacteria.

Cholesterol Buster

Bunch of Parsley
Bunch of Spinach
(6) Carrots
(1) Half Garlic Clove
(2) Large Slices of Pineapple

This juice combination contains Vitamin C which lowers Cholesterol. The Spinach and Carrots are excellent sources of Vitamin E which improves circulation. The Parsley contains Vitamin C, Magnesium and Potassium very helpful in lowering Cholesterol levels.

Note Bunch together Parsley, Spinach and Garlic. Push through with Carrots. Don't forget to remove Carrot Tops.

Common Cold Relief

(6) Carrots
Handful of Parsley
(1) Garlic Clove
(3) Stalks of Celery
(1) Tomato

The nutrients found in this juice are Beta Carotene, Vitamin C and Zinc. This juice combination is good for the immune system. It gets rid of bacteria and is anti-viral.

Note Push through Parsley and Garlic with Carrots to make sure you get the constituents of both.

Cancer Tonic

(1) Whole Cabbage
(1) Apple
(4) Stalks of Celery

Cancer is a very serious condition, and because it is you must change your dietary habits completely. If you have

Cancer I suggest drinking the above juice combination at least (4) times a day or more according to how developed the Cancer is. You also need too greatly increase your intake of fresh organic raw fruits and vegetables. You must also eliminate all animal protein! Drink big glasses of this juice combination.

High Blood Pressure Relief Tonic

(1) Apple
(6) Carrots (remove tops)
Bunch/Handful of Spinach
(8) Strawberries
Bunch/Handful of Parsley
(2) Garlic Cloves

Push through Spinach, Parsley, Strawberries and Garlic with Carrots. This juice combination is a rich source of Magnesium and Calcium. This combination lowers your blood pressure.

Hypoglycemia Drink

(5) Kale Leaves
Bunch of Spinach
(6) Carrots (remove tops)
(1) Apple
(1) Large Slice Pineapple

This juice combination contains Chromium which helps to regulate insulin levels. This combination also includes Magnanese which helps in Glucose Metabolism.

Infection Relief Juice

Bunch of Parsley
Bunch of Spinach
1 Half Lemon
1 Half Apple
(6) Carrots
(1) Large Slice of Pineapple
Remove the seeds of the Lemon.

This juice combination contains Zinc, Vitamin C, Beta Carotene, Sodium and Potassium. All fight the killer cells.

Bedtime Tonic

(5) Stalks Celery
Bunch of Parsley
(1) Apple
(2) Stalks of Asparagus
(1) Tomato
(1) Large Slice of Pineapple

This combination contains Niacin, Magnesium, B6, Calcium and Folate. This juice combination helps you sleep because of the sleep inducing chemical Serotonin. This juice combination also helps your muscles to relax.
Note Push through Parsley with Celery

Menstrual Relief Tonic

(6) Carrots (tops removed)
Bunch of Parsley
(2) Stalks Broccoli
(2) Kale Leaves
(1) Apple
(1) Slice Pineapple

This juice combination contains Iron which aids in decreasing excessive Menstrual bleeding and cramping. This juice combination contains Vitamin C which reduces bleeding. It also contains Vitamin K (Chlorophyll) which reduces bleeding. It also contains Bromelain from the Pineapple which has anti-inflammatory properties.

Severe Headache Juice (Migraines)

(4) Stalks Celery
(6) Carrots (tops removed)
Bunch of Parsley
Bunch of Spinach
1 Half Inch Slice of Ginger Root

This juicing combination is for the worst type of headache, the Migraine. This juicing combination contains Magnesium which relaxes the muscles in your head.

Push through Parsley and Spinach with Carrots

Prostate Relief Juice

Bunch of Parsley
(6) Carrots (tops removed)
(2) Kale Leaves
Bunch of Spinach
(1) Large Tomato

In this juice combination the Parsley and Carrots contain Zinc which reduces the size of the Prostate and relieves symptoms in various men. The Kale and the Spinach contain B6 that is a good partner of Zinc. It helps in combination with Zinc to reduce Prolactin levels. I also recommend eating Pumpkin seeds which is a great source of Zinc and required fatty acids. Also take Flaxseed Oil (2) times a day because this is also a great help for the Prostate.

More About The Prostate

Many men develop Prostate Cancer here in the United States and around the world each year. If not treated early enough it can become deadly. The Physicians' Health Study and the European Prospective Investigation in Cancer and Nutrition say that men who drink lots of milk have a higher risk of Prostate Cancer.

It said that men who drink more than 600 mg. of Calcium from dairy products (2) 8-ounce glasses of milk had a significant 32% increased risk of Prostate Cancer. This was compared to men who consumed less than 150 mg. of Calcium from dairy products. If you need Calcium there are plant sources of Calcium. Green and Orange foods and dark *leafy greens are a great source. Nuts are also a great source of Calcium along with sesame seeds found in Tahini.*

Psoriasis Relief Tonic

(6) Carrots (tops removed)
(1) Beet
1 Half Apple
(2) Kale Leaves
Bunch of Parsley
(1) Orange (remove peel and seeds)

In this juicing combination the Carrots and Parsley contain Zinc which produces healthy looking skin. The Beet is a powerful detoxifier and cleanser. Kale and the Carrot are also great sources of Beta Carotene which contain Vitamin A and help in new skin growth. The Orange contains Selenium which decreases inflammatory problems.

Ulcer Tonic Juice

(2) Stalks Celery
(1) Half Cabbage
(1) Apple

The Cabbage and the Celery contain powerful Ulcer healing properties. I use the Apple as a sweetener, but it also has healing properties with the Pectin which is contained in the Apple. The nutrients found in these (3) healing vegetables are Zinc, Vitamin E and C.

Twisted Juice (Varicose Veins)

(6) Carrots (tops removed)
(3) Stalks Celery
Bunch of Parsley
1 Large Slice of Pineapple
(4) Kale Leaves
(1) Apple
(2) Cloves Garlic
1 Fourth Cantaloupe

In this juice combination the Carrots, Parsley and Kale contain Beta Carotene which is a healing ingredient. Celery reduces inflammation. The Pineapple contains Bromelain which helps prevent the formation of blood clots. The Apple is a great immune booster. The Garlic reduces the risk of blocked arteries. Cantaloupe decreases the risk of heart attack, associated in blood clots with varicose veins.

Gout Relief Tonic

(10) Cherries (remove pits)
(10) Strawberries (firm)
(4) Kale Leaves
Bunch of Wheat Grass
(2) Apples
(3) Stalks Celery
(1) Slice of Pineapple
(1) Slice of Cantaloupe
Gout is a result of too much Uric Acid in your system. This is caused by you eating too many foods of animal origin.

This results in a very high level of this Uric Acid. This in turn causes the Uric Acid to crystallize in your joints which causes swelling and strong pain in your feet or ankles. It can also cause you to have chills and fever. The Cherries, Wheat Grass, Apple, Cantaloupe and Kale contain Vitamin C which neutralizes Uric Acid. The Celery and Pineapple reduce the inflammation.

Remembering Juice (Alzheimers)

(2) Beets
(5) Carrots
(2) Apples
Bunch Of Spinach
(2) Stalks Celery
(2) Kale Leaves

The Beets in this juice combination are high in Vitamin A which strengthens and nourishes the Liver. Beets also contain Choline from Acetylcholine which is a brain chemical that plays an important role in reasoning and cognition. Beets are also a good source of Potassium. The Carrots and Beets are high in Beta Carotene which promotes mental functioning. The Apples also contain Beta Carotene. The Spinach is rich in iron and Beta Carotene and is a great detoxifier. Spinach is also good for anemia because of its iron content. The Kale is high in Calcium. The celery reduces inflammation. This juice is good for helping prevent Dementia and Alzheimers, which result from Free Radicals and inflammation of brain tissue. I also recommend eating Lentils, Mung Beans and Brazil Nuts which contain Choline.

Bronchitis Juice

(6) Carrots (tops removed)
(2) Cloves of Garlic
(1) Lemon (remove seeds)
Bunch of Spinach
An Eighth Teaspoon of Cayenne Pepper

This juice combination is great for fighting infection. It is great for dissolving mucus. It also stimulates the immune system. This juice combination is good for coughs, colds and the flu.

Diabetic Tonic

(3) Artichokes
(2) Stalks Broccoli
Bunch of Parsley
1 Fourth Head of Fennel
(10) String Beans

This juice combination helps maintain normal blood sugar levels. It's rich in Vitamin E and Phytonutrients. This juice is also good for the kidneys. String Beans contain elements which furnish the ingredients for natural insulin. This is a great juice for Diabetics.

Gall Stone Eliminator Juice

1 Half Lemon (remove seeds)
(5) Radishes
(4) Tomatoes
(8) Carrots
(2) Stalks Celery
Bunch of Parsley
(1) Apple

This juice combination is of great benefit for Gallstones because it is a diuretic. It cleanses the liver and digestive track and reduces inflammation. Finally, it is highly important if you have problems with Gallstones to reduce your intake of animal protein.

Kidney Stone Eliminator Juice

(4) Carrots (remove tops)
(2) Apples
(12) Asparagus Spears
(2) Stalks Broccoli
(2) Cloves Garlic

This juice combination is good for flushing and removing Kidney Stones from the body. This juice is good for the digestive track because it is a diuretic. It promotes healing and is rich in Vitamin E. It is great in fighting infection, and gets rid of poisons from the body.

Herpes Simplex Booster

Bunch of Spinach
Bunch of Parsley
(2) Apples
(2) Cloves Garlic
(4) Stalks Celery
(6) Carrots (remove tops)

This juicing combination is great for a weak Immune System. The juices in this combination help strengthen the Immune System to fight infection. This juice combination is highly effective in fighting skin infections. It is rich in vitamins, minerals and other nutrients. *Push Spinach and Parsley through with Carrots*

Indigestion Relief Juice

(1) Squash
(2) Sweet Potatoes
(2) Large Slices of Pineapple
(1) Half Teaspoon of Cayenne Pepper
(6) Carrots

The Bromelain in the Pineapple is great for indigestion, as well as the other juices.

Lupus Tonic

(2) Apples
(4) Stalks Broccoli
1 Fourth Head of Cabbage
1 Fourth Head of Cauliflower
1 Half Lemon (remove seeds)

This juice combination is a good source of Choline. Choline is a brain chemical needed for anyone with Lupus. Choline is responsible for reasoning and cognition. Choline is high in Vitamin E which is good for soft tissue. This juice combination inhibits the development of harmful chemical carcinogens within the body. This juice combination is anti-inflammatory thus promoting healing. This juice is high in Endoles, a powerful Cancer fighting agent. This juice is an immune builder and is anti-bacterial.

Multiple Sclerosis Juicer

(10) Carrots (remove tops)
(2) Beets
(2) Apples
Bunch of Spinach
(4) Kale Leaves

This juice combination is a great immune booster. It's an antioxidant, an antiseptic and anti-bacterial. It's rich in Vitamin A, B, and C. It's rich in the minerals Iron, Calcium, Potassium and Sodium. This juice is also high in levels of Folate which is good for the Spinal Cord, especially for a condition such as Multiple Sclerosis.

*Push Kale and Spinach through with Carrots.

Special Bonus Section

Health authorities, doctors, etc. say eat (5) fruits and vegetables to get all of your intake of vitamins and minerals. Well, if you juice, you are getting the liquid, the concentrated form of these fruits and vegetables. I call it "Liquid Gold." This "Liquid Gold" goes directly into your bloodstream. It goes into your body instantly! This juice is full of Hydrogen Ions an antioxidant, a Free Radical fighter.

Juicing is a power source of antioxidant power that fights disease and aging. It gives you energy and makes you feel good. It makes you feel like you're going back to your youth.

The main reason most peoples bodies breakdown when they get older is because of lack of exercise and proper nutrition. If you do not take in the proper nutrition your body can still breakdown even if you exercise.

Over 10 years ago a well known fitness expert fell dead with a Heart Attack while running. That's where proper nutrition comes in. If you don't eat the right foods are drink the right drinks, then your arteries can still clog up and you can die of a Heart Attack. This also goes for any other life ending condition as well.

Doctors treat symptoms with drugs. They tell their patients that they must stay on these drugs for the remainder of their life. Drugs have never healed anyone of any condition! Your body has the power to heal itself. Drugs can only reduce symptoms.

When we eat "Live Food" (food not cooked) our bodies then get the nourishment to produce a healthy body. When we cook these "Live Foods" we destroy the "Life Giving Enzymes." The heat in the cooking process makes this a "Dead Food." You only have the key to good health!

EWG, The Environmental Working Group not long ago published a study of pesticide concentration in foods in the Shoppers Guide to pesticides in April, 2009. (www.foodnews. org)

EWG said that people who eat the 12 most contaminated fruits and vegetables consume an average of 10 pesticides a day. Those who ate the 15 least contaminated conventionally grown fruits and vegetables ingest fewer than 2 pesticides daily. (page 9) Two (2) pesticides daily is too much. That's why it's important for you too eat Organic grown fruits and vegetables.

Starting on the next pages are my special juicing combinations. These are juices that are really healthy, and ones I enjoy. I hope you will too!

Morning Power Juice

(2) & 1 Fourth Quarter Cantaloupe & Rind
(1) & 1 Fourth Watermelon & Rind
(1) Bunch of Spinach
(1) Half Pear
(1) Apple
(2) Slices Pineapple
(2) 1 Fourth Quarter Lemon (remove seeds)
(1) Stalk Broccoli
(12) Red Grapes
(8) Large Carrots

This makes 36 ounces of juice that is loaded with vitamins and life giving nutrients. Drink all and rejuvenate.

*Why am I juicing the Cantaloupe and Watermelon Rinds? The Rinds are packed with powerful health strengthening enzymes, vitamins and Phytonutrients. These skins have significant illness curing, disease fighting nutrients.

Lemon Zest

(2) Lemons
Bunch of Spinach
Bunch of Parsley
(8) Large Carrots
(1) Pear
(4) Large Chunks Pineapple

Remove the seeds of the Lemon.

Tomato Surprise

(2) Large Tomatoes
(1) Half Pear
(1) Half Lemon
(1) Half Sweet Potato
(10) Carrots
(2) Slices Pineapple

Remove seeds of the Lemon.

Cantaloupe/Pineapple Express

(2) Large Slices Cantaloupe
(1) Half Pear
(3) Large One Half Slices Pineapple

Bunch of Spinach

"Tastes Great"

Peachy

(1) Half Lemon
(3) Whole Peaches (remove pits)
(1) Apple
(1) Slice Pineapple
Remove seeds of the Lemon.

Wowwwh!

Grape Power Punch

(1) Half Lemon
Bunch of Parsley
(2) Apples
(10) Red Grapes

Remove seeds of the Lemon.

umm,umm, good!

Green Power

(1) Large Slice Pineapple
(2) Apples
(4) Strawberries (firm)
(1) Stalk of Broccoli
(1) Fourth Lemon
(4) Stalks of Kale
Bunch of Parsley
Bunch f Spinach
(2) Carrots
Remove the seeds of the Lemon.

*Push Kale, Parsley and Spinach through with Carrots.

The Red One

(1) Half Beet
(1) Fourth Lemon
(2) Apples
(1) Slice of Watermelon Rind
(6) Carrots
Remove seeds of the Lemon.

The Beet dominates this juice. It's good for your Liver.

Zinger

(1) Half Ginger Root
(1) Apple
(8) Strawberries
(6) Carrots
(1) Half Lemon (remove seeds)

One of my favorite juices very zestful.

Strawberry Surprise

Bunch of Parsley
(1) Half Lemon (remove seeds)
(1) Apple
(1) Slice of Sweet Potato
(2) Carrots
(10) Strawberries (firm)

My Oh My, That's good!

Pectin Power

(2) Apples (Golden Delicious)
(1) Half Lemon
Bunch of Parsley
(1) Slice of Pineapple
(6) Carrots
Remove seeds of the Lemon.

Another Great Tasting Juice!

Thumbs Up Juice

(6) Carrots
Bunch of Spinach
Bunch of Parsley
(1) Tomato
(1) Pear
(1) Apple
(1) Lemon
(1) Slice of Pineapple
(1) Stalk Broccoli
(1) Slice of Watermelon Rind
Remove seeds of the Lemon.
This Is A Vitamin Packed Power Juice. Enjoy!

Vitamin Power

(8) Carrots
Bunch of Spinach
Bunch of Parsley
(1) Tomato
(8) Grapes (red)
(2) Stalks Broccoli
(1) Apple
(1) Slice Pineapple
(1) Fourth Beet

When You Speak Of Vitamins This Is A Superior Vitamin Enriched Juice.

Tootie Fruitie

(15) Strawberries (firm)
(15) Grapes (red)
(2) Apples
(15) Blueberries (firm)
(2) Large Slices Pineapple
(1) Half Lemon (remove seeds)

A Great Combination of Fruits, a Fantastic Taste!

Intestinal Relief Juice (Constipation)

(3) Apples
(3) Handfuls of Spinach

This works because the Pectin in Apples mix with the Oxalic Acid in Spinach and produce a powerful internal cleansing process. This juice combination sticks to and infiltrates the walls of the Colon getting rid of fecal matter that has accumulated over a period of time. (weeks, months, possibly years) Drink this juice once a day for 5 days. You'll feel much better too. (Use Golden Delicious or McIntosh Apples)

ABOUT THE AUTHOR

In 1996, I began juicing because of a tremendous health scare I had. Shortly thereafter, I saw an infomercial on television with the Original Juice Man, Jay Kordich. Jay Kordich survived and overcame a life threatening illness because of juicing. He juiced a daily regiment of organic carrot and apple juice. While watching the infomercial, Mr. Kordich was advertising his Juice Man Juicer and talked about the power of juicing. I started juicing a daily regiment of organic carrot, apple, spinach, parsley, beet and pineapple juice. I also eliminated animal protein, I lost 30 pounds in a month. The condition I had disappeared in no time. I want you too know that you too can overcome illness and disease through juicing. I want you too know that you can be well again. I want you too know that it's not too late to start juicing now.

The Juicing Man, Fred L. Gist

Pineapple Cabbage Blend

1 Cabbage
2 slices of Pineapple
1 half Lemon
1 Apple
1 Orange
Remove the seeds of the Lemon.
This is a sweeter mixture of the Cancer tonic.

Digestion

Digestion is very important to your overall health. If toxins are in your system, they will limit your ability to achieve great health. You have to eat many more cleansing foods, like Organic raw whole foods in the forms of fruits and vegetables.

Juicing grasses like Wheat Grass is a significant way to cleanse your internal organs. Juicing this grass will give you the vital nutrients to rid your digestive system of these toxins.

Fiber

I wanted to also talk briefly about the importance of getting Fiber into your system. I eat about a cup full of Fiber each time I juice. The Fiber or pulp from the raw fruits and vegetables you juice is great for the intestinal tract. This pulp plays an important role in preventing colon cancer. It's also good to prevent constipation. I also eat lots of raw organic fruits and vegetables each week that's full of this pulp.

FINAL THOUGHTS

You may feel great. You may look great. You may have no symptoms of illness or disease. That's great. It's still very important to start juicing. Juicing as I mentioned earlier, has results just like if you have taken a laxative.

Your body is eliminating toxins, free radicals out of your body. Most people don't know that most of your illness and disease start because you have an unhealthy colon. Fecal matter has built up over a period of time. This fecal matter lies in your colon dormant, and then causes other problems to arise in your body over a matter of time.

When you juice organic fruits and vegetables you develop a much healthier colon. You develop healthier cells. Your body fights off these free radials through juicing. Juicing is the healthiest thing you can do for your body.

The Juicing Man, Fred L. Gist

4 THINGS TO HELP YOU LIVE LONGER

1. Walk at least 30 minutes a day. There are great physical and healthy benefits in this exercise. If you jog or do more strenuous exercise this benefits you more.

2. Try to reach your optimal weight. The way you know you have done this is this. If you are 5'8 inches tall then you are 68 inches high. You now want to divide this by 2. This will give you 34 inches which is your waist size. This is where you want to be. This helps keep the added stress off of your body by lowering your blood pressure and more.

3. Go to bed earlier. Lack of sleep increases heart disease, diabetes, and obesity. Studies have shown that 7 to 8 hours of sleep is ideal to help you live longer.

4. Juice, eat organic fruits and vegetables. Juice and eat the different colors of the organic fruit and vegetable rainbow like the reds, greens, yellows, purples, and blues. These colorful, vibrant organic fruits and vegetables are full of powerful antioxidants that fight off illness and disease.

REFERENCES

1. Max Gerson, A Cancer Therapy, results of fifty cases
2. Dr. Norman Walker, Fresh Vegetable and Fruit Juices
3. Jay Kordick, The Original Juice Man
4. Dr. George Malkmus, Hallelujah Acres
5. Dr. Lee W. Wattenburg, Department of Laboratory Medicine and Pathology, University of Minnesota
6. Physicians Health Study, The European Prospective Investigation in Cancer and Nutrition
7. The Environmental Working Group, www.foodnews.org
8. Jack Lalane, The Jack Lalane Power Juicer

CHANGE YOUR EATING HABITS TO BECOME WELL AGAIN

To get well, to overcome any illness or disease starts with you completely changing your diet. You must eliminate fried foods, fatty foods, salt, and sugar. You must eliminate carbohydrates, which your body converts to sugar. If you smoke or drink, then stop.

You should start an exercise program, and greatly increase your intake of organic fruits and vegetable juices. You should also eat lots of fresh organic raw fruits and vegetables. This is the only way you can completely heal your body.

The Juicing Man, Fred L. Gist

WASHING YOUR ORGANIC FRUITS AND VEGETABLES

Always wash your Organic Fruits and Vegetables to remove any dirt. Wash these fruits and vegetables in warm water and check to make sure all dirt is removed. It's important to do this because I've found that some Organic grocery stores do not wash their Organic Fruits and Vegetables well. Lots of time they just don't probably have the time.

BENEFITS OF USING A JUICER

Juicing through a juicer is an excellent way to obtain nutritional values from a large amount of Organic fruits and vegetables. This prevents you from having to eat large amounts of these same Organic fruits and vegetables. It's much easier to juice than to try too eat large amounts of Organic fruits and vegetables to obtain nutritional benefits.

WHAT JUICER DO I USE

I use two different juicers, the Jack Lalane Power Juicer and the Juiceman Jr. I love both these juicers because of the wide opening for the fruits and vegetables. You can put a small apple in both openings. You don't have to cut the smaller fruits and vegetables as you would with more expensive juicers. Both juicers also have the power you need.

Both juicers also produce more juice than less expensive juicers. You can purchase the Jack Lalane Power Juicer with warranty on line for around 100.00 dollars. You can also purchase the Jack Lalane Power Juicer at Walmart for around 100.00 also. You can purchase the Juiceman Jr. which has two different speeds for around 90.00 dollars at Walmart.

VITAMIN E

One nutrient that has been widely studied over the years is Vitamin E. Vitamin E has been shown to boost healthy functioning of the immune system.

Research suggests that Vitamin E enhances the immune system and protects it against damage from free radicals. The food sources you can get Vitamin E from are nuts, seeds, grains and wheat germ. The juice of green leafy vegetables such as Spinach, Kale and Swiss Chard are most beneficial.

Sulfur, Beta Carotene and Cancer

In recent years studies have shown that certain foods do help prevent and reverse certain kinds of cancer. As mentioned earlier the juice of the Cabbage is one. Sulfur compounds found in Cabbage stimulate the activity of liver enzymes that detoxify carcinogens. This sulfur compound is also found in garlic.

Beta Carotene which contains Vitamin A is found in many vegetables and fruits like Carrots, Cantaloupe, Broccoli, Sweet Potatoes and Pumpkin to name a few. Juicing and eating many different kinds of fruits and vegetables is the key in preventing and overcoming cancer. You also must cut down your intake of saturated fats and eat healthy amounts of fiber.

Organic

Organic is a term used to describe food grown without the use of chemicals, pesticides and fertilizers. All foods that say Organic are certified by the United States Department of

Agriculture. These Organic foods are then held to very high standards.

There are no antibiotics or hormones used with Organic grown foods. All feed fed to animals is 100 percent Organic feed. There are no unnatural substances used in the soil. The soil used in Organic farming is healthy soil.

Finally, Organic foods are far more expensive, but switching to them is worth your health.

Exercise

Do some type of exercise and reap rewards that come with exercise. The bonus can come at the end of your life with more added years. Exercise will help bring back your vitality and rejuvenate your body. When you don't exercise you can gain weight that becomes dangerous to your body. If you don't exercise the body will age faster.

Exercise makes your heart pump more oxygen-rich blood with less effort. This keeps you from getting tired as quickly if you didn't exercise. Exercise also helps to lower blood pressure and also normalizes blood sugar.

Exercise increases the mass and strength of your bones and the flexibility of your joints. Exercise helps to fight off diseases by boosting the immune system. Exercise helps you shed weight and stay trim. You eat less and also you are more mentally alert. I can attest to the benefits of exercise. I exercise regularly and along with juicing I have no ailments of any kind.

The Juicing Man, Fred L. Gist

Vitamin D

An important vitamin that has tremendous health benefits for your immune system is Vitamin D. Most people are deficient in this very important vitamin.

Vitamin D helps facilitate the absorption of calcium in the bloodstream and plays a very important role in maintaining bone density. Some people weighing more than 180 pounds may require higher doses of Vitamin D. Leading experts recommend 2,000 -7,000 IU of this vitamin per day.

Studies have shown that vitamin D has a huge impact in boosting your immune system. Older people are at risk for cognitive impairment when they lack sufficient Vitamin D.

The lack of sufficient Vitamin D in older adults is associated with frailty among them as well. There is also supporting evidence that sufficient Vitamin D levels may help prevent cognitive decline and Alzheimers' disease. Everyone from young adults to older adults must take sufficient amounts of Vitamin D too help maintain a healthy immune system.

Coconut Oil

Coconut Oil is very nutritious and rich in minerals and vitamins. It has many health benefits and has been used traditionally among Pacific and Asian people. The Coconut Palm is called the Tree of Life by people who live on the Pacific Islands.

The Coconut Palm or Tree is called the Tree of Life because it is valued highly by these people as a source of food and medicine. Recently modern science has found secrets to the amazing healing powers of the coconut.

Around the planet, oil of the Coconut is used to treat many health problems. Some of these health problems are the flu, constipation, burns, asthma, kidney stones, painful menstruation, rashes, tumors, gonorrhea, tuberculosis, and more.

Coconut Oil is great for your skin because it penetrates into the deepest layers keeping your skin strong and supple. It also reduces fine lines and wrinkles, and makes the skin smoother.

Cayenne Pepper

I love Cayenne Pepper. I put it on chicken, fish, pork chops and other meats. I put it on vegetables, rice, potatoes, spaghetti and other starches. It's good for you. It improves your circulation. It's good to help fight off colds. It's good for sinus problems and it's good for your heart.

Cayenne Pepper has been known to stop heart attacks. It removes plaque from your arteries. It lowers cholesterol. It has been scientifically proven to kill prostate cancer cells. It improves your overall health. I buy Cayenne Pepper from local health food stores where it comes as a bulk item.

Cayenne Pepper comes in different degrees as far as how hot it is. I recommend you get the mildest, unless you like it hotter.

Unfiltered Apple Cider Vinegar

In my juicing you notice that I use a lot of apples. Of course you have heard the saying, An Apple a Day Keeps the Doctor Away. Apples are high in pectin and other power vitamins and minerals. Apples are high in antioxidant power that fight off free radicals. Apple Cider Vinegar processed from the apple has been used as a medicine and food.

The Father of Modern Medicine, Hippocrates used Apple Cider Vinegar mixed with honey. Apple Cider Vinegar has been used to treat many ailments like Diabetes, Warts, Gout and Acid Reflux to name a few. You can buy this Unfiltered Apple Cider Vinegar from a health food store.

Olive Oil

Olive Oil is full of antioxidants. I cook in Olive Oil. I put it over my salads. Olive Oil is high in monounsaturated fat, a very safe fatty acid. Olive Oil protects your heart from heart disease.

Olive Oil raises the good cholesterol level HDL, and controls LDL bad cholesterol. Olive Oil has the largest amount of monounsaturated fat of any oil. Extra Virgin Olive Oil also contains higher levels of the antioxidant Vitamin E.

Would you like to see your manuscript become a book?

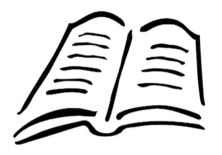

If you are interested in becoming a PublishAmerica author, please submit your manuscript for possible publication to us at:

acquisitions@publishamerica.com

You may also mail in your manuscript to:

**PublishAmerica
PO Box 151
Frederick, MD 21705**

We also offer free graphics for Children's Picture Books!

---

www.publishamerica.com

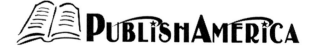

CPSIA information can be obtained at www.ICGtesting.com
Printed in the USA
LVOW05*0859200514

386557LV00005B/14/P

9 781462 649419